DISCLAIMER/LEGAL NOTICES

Publisher:

New Dreams, Colors and Faces.

Email: NDCFace@gmail.com

Become A Nurse,

LVN OR LPN

in 12 Months or Less!

A Career Guide for:
Immigrants, Certified Nurse Aides, Home Health Aides, Babysitters and You!

Dedication

Career Changers Who Dare to Become Nurses!

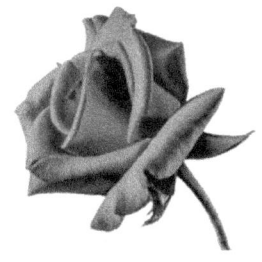

This Book Belongs To

Name:

Date:

Thank You

The delivery of healthcare in America is facilitated by many professionals including **State Boards of Nursing, Nurses**, **Certified Nurse Aides,** Corporate investors, Insurance companies, Pharmaceutical companies, **Doctors,** Administrators, Social Workers, Physician Assistants**, Physical Therapists,** PT Aides, Occupational Therapists, OT Aides, Speech Therapists, Activities Coordinators, **Dietary Managers**, Diagnostic/Lab Technicians, **Pharmacists,** Delivery services, **Hospitality Staff,** Dietary Aides, Cooks, Dishwashers, Maintenance Managers, Plumbers, Electricians, Hairdressers, Barbers**, EMS/Transport/Fire/Law Enforcement Services**, Funeral Homes and **Med Aides.**

"Thank you" for serving with empathy and integrity!

Table of Contents

ACKNOWLEDGEMENTS

NOTES

Special Message

Thank you for reading about my LVN/LPN experience and trusting me to guide you to a similar State Approved school. My goal is to **prepare you with the right information before you waste valuable time and money on a program that may not be the 'right fit' for you and to help you avoid fake schools!**

Recently an investigation by several states, titled *"Operation Nightingale"*, discovered fake nurses working in various states with fake nursing diplomas and transcripts bought from several accredited Florida schools (Texas Board of Nursing Bulletin, p. 1, April 2023).

How did that happen? For one thing, it is important to find a school that will teach you nursing theory and make it mandatory that you attend all your clinical classes. You will need to read the rest of this book to know more about how to protect your investment of time and money!

At present, I have two (2) questions for you. Who are you, and how would you describe yourself? The answers you provide determine how you prepare to get into an Approved LVN/LPN school.

Fortunately, I am a working nurse today because I used my dissatisfaction about my former job conditions to fuel me to take the necessary steps to attend nursing school. I hope after you read my book, you will be inspired to take positive steps and go to a great nursing school!

I am writing this book with an unapologetic bias towards Certified Nurse's Aides (CNAs) because I was one! I need CNAs to know, that I know how it feels to be cleaning, feeding, and consoling sick patients—under challenging workloads! Therefore, I am proud to finally write a book that will show CNAs the pathway or 'great escape', to upgrade their skills to become nurses!

Let us talk about nursing facts. According to the United States Department of Labor, there is a nursing shortage of an estimated two hundred, seventy-five thousand (275,000) nurses (**https://www.dol.gov).** Until 2030, all types of nurses, including LVNs/LPNs will continue to be in high demand! We will always need nurses if life on this planet continues to exist!

Are you ready to fill one of those 275,000 vacancies by adding more value to your work skills? My dear reader, notice I did not say "add more value to you the person" because you the person is not about a nursing title, since you are created in the likeness of your Creator/God! If you lost all your titles today, you would remain a fabulous, creative person with the inner creativity to solve your own problems!

Therefore, if your answer is "yes to nursing school", then my book contains all the information you will need to get mentally, financially, emotionally, physically, and spiritually **prepared to seek out a program that meets your needs and lifestyle!**

Which title is more valuable-RN or LVN/LPN?

At present, **the gold standard for nursing education is a Registered Nurse program, preferably at the bachelor's level,** and **accredited** by one of the reputable accreditation nursing agencies, in the United States of America. For instance, the Accreditation Commission for Education in Nursing (ACEN) oversees all educational nursing levels: Practical Nursing programs/L.P.N. or L.V.N., diploma, associate's, bachelor's, master's, and doctoral degrees.

Other students may consider their **silver standard** in nursing as a two (2) year **Associate's, R.N. program**. However, there are some prospective LVNs/LPNS who may view their future licenses **as their 'bronze' medals to a brighter future! While I agree with the above views on nursing education, I see the LVN/LPN position as a "learning gold mine" and a "come up" to help my patients and advance my own quality of life!**

Why did I write this book?

I wanted to answer the following **four (4) questions:**

- "How can you get into an L.V.N./L.P.N. program?

- Which school should you go to?
- Where can you get money to pay for school?
- What were my (the author's) strategies to study and pass all school assignments and exams?"

The answers to the top three (3) questions will be answered in this first book. The last question will be answered in a follow-up book titled **"Success Strategies for L.V.N./L.P.N. School and passing your License Exam on the first try!"** The second book will be out sometime in 2023 wherever books are sold in the U.S.A.

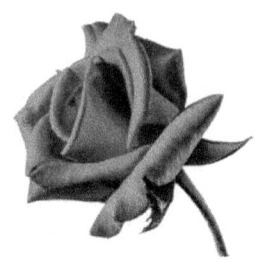

PART ONE

Mental Preparation

Chapter 1
You and Nursing

leave it up to you to figure out how you are going to sort out logical ways to save your money to go to nursing school. However, I will offer my own suggestions on how to do so in the last chapter. This section is about mental preparation, with specific details to help you create strategies on how to apply to an L.V.N./L.P.N. school.

First, I would like you to have a vision or clear picture in your mind about the way you will use your education upon completion of school. If you can "see it" or imagine being a nursing student, **then you can write your vision on paper.** Second, you **must believe it in your mind**, and your beliefs will build a strong desire within you to **take actions to achieve your goal within the next year or two (2) years!**

Also, you will need a small support system of one (1) or two (2) individuals as you plan to go to nursing school. I built inner strength from a few friends who encouraged me, when I decided during Covid 19, to step away from a BSN/RN program to focus on a lower, basic, LVN/LPN program!

Life had handed me some proverbial lemons or imbalance, and I made myself a tall glass of life's best, proverbial 'lemonade' or an orderly, manageable way to finish nursing school! Today, I am happy I did a short, quick program that allowed me to graduate faster to be able to work. Some students in the BSN RN program decided against my choice and chose to leave school for the same job and circumstances they had left behind!

You may face a similar scenario too when you decide to move from C.N.A. to attend an L.V.N./L.P.N. school. Some people may not share your dream and may even discourage you from your conviction that you can overcome all obstacles to become a nurse! Your job is to focus on the encouragement in this book and proceed!

Also, your choice of an L.V.N./L.P.N. career will allow you to be available to pursue other interests, such as entrepreneurial activities. To this end, **a side hustle for example, selling a service or a product, is essential to one's post pandemic strategies to create financial stability against the unexpected, instability of our economy,** for examples: inflation with high food, gas prices and future pandemics.

Who is an LVN/LPN?

Licensed professional nurses have titles, such as: L.V.N./L.P.N., R.N., and APRN or NP and DNP. Each letter in those titles means something. This book is for you, if you would like to pursue a Licensed Vocational Nurse or Practical Nurse (L.V.N./L.P.N.) education. Concisely, **all nurses are licensed professionals, whatever their titles!**

Beginner nurses are referred to as Vocational or Practical nurses in the United States of America, it depends on your location. I live in the South, so I am a Licensed Vocational Nurse (L.V.N.). Where do you live? Figure out what title you will be called. I know on the East Coast, for example, in New York and New Jersey, the title is Licensed Practical Nurse (L.P.N.). **The time will come when you shall say, "I am a Licensed Professional Nurse."**

The above paragraph is important to keep in mind because there are people who may attempt to make you feel you are of lesser value as an L.V.N./L.P.N. compared to a Registered Nurse (R.N.). **You are valuable as a person, and you will add more value to your work skills when you upgrade them to become a wise, basic nurse! Licensed Vocational Nurses (LVNs/LPNs) are much appreciated by both employers and the patients they care for, especially in this nursing shortage!**

RN or LVN, which is better for Your Situation?

Let us have a big picture view of what it means to become a nursing student and then a nurse, so that you can plan your next step towards getting admitted into school.

If you need proof of your potential value, take a working L.V.N./L.P.N. as an example, especially those who have been in the field for at least two (2) years- who are employed and make over $50,000 annually!

It **is better to gain financial stability on an L.V.N./L.P.N. salary, with little or no school debt, before rushing for another title, that one may not be able to fund** at a specific stage of one's life. Goals require planning, time, and money, and you need all three (3) ingredients to invest in a good L.V.N./L.P.N. or an R.N. school.

What is your current life's stage and age? Based on your age, you will experience unique needs as you grow, especially if you are beyond childbearing age. Remember whatever your life's stage you will need: shelter-a house or apartment, clothes, food, money to pay your bills, education (self-education/this book, and formal/nursing school), and a support system of people who care about you!

Likewise, when you become a new nurse, it is important to take your time to become a clinically capable and time conscientious nurse. **Therefore, I need you to see the employment road ahead based on your lifestyle, age, personal likes, and dislikes -for example, certain clinical tasks, and have a plan to focus on your strengths.** Remember, the Registered Nurse option gives you better career options that may be suited to your temperament and career goals. **The question is which of** the two (2) titles can you afford and how much time will it take you to get in and out of school, faster?

Some students may not choose L.V.N./L.P.N. programs because they would prefer to work in settings which require a higher level of education such as a Bachelor of Science in Nursing/RN program, and work alongside higher-level thinkers in top tier hospitals. I agree one hundred percent (100%) with that opinion because lower-level thinkers tend to drain one's energy, and some are not team oriented! You went to school to be your best so stick with those who are about building positive relationships and uplifting the nursing profession.

Therefore, once you get licensed do not stay at an L.V.N./L.P.N. level where you are limited to mostly clinical bedside nursing, in nursing homes. Nursing is a broad field with many non-clinical jobs such as informatics, Nurse Manager, Nurse Instructor, and many other positions that are outside the scope of this basic book.

However, one is not to despise his or her day of small beginnings with an L.V.N./L.P.N. title, that small title can be used as your key to open another door to the goal of becoming a Registered Nurse (R.N.) or opening a small business to sell a service! For example, research the many businesses owned by competent and qualified nurses, from LVN to NP level.

What am I doing with the little that God gave me to start off? I am writing a book to help you to get into school and later you too can tell your own story on your way out by writing the book you have been dreaming about! Therefore, think outside the traditional, nursing box of jobs!

The Post pandemic, global job market is about using all available opportunities for any worker to flip their education to earn a living! Nursing knowledge is no exception to this rule, so do not wait until you get a higher nursing education to "shake things up" to make your coins! While others argue about titles, use what you know along life's path to help you thrive in nursing school and beyond!

Employee or Independent Contractor

This conversation is necessary after you graduate, but I placed it here, for those of you who are figuring out the job landscape before you apply to a school. You may choose to be an employee or a self-employed nurse if your personality, stage of life, temperament is suited to one type, rather than the other types of employment, such as entrepreneurs or owners of businesses.

Professional nurses including LVNs/LPNs are qualified and suited to be entrepreneurs, based on their level of knowledge, skills, and business goals. **You may need to get away from the traditional mindset that being an** employee is more stable and prestigious than having your own business—especially when America is going through cyclical recessions every seven (7) years or so!

Also, employee-nurses can be either Full Time, Part Time, or PRN. The first position qualifies for benefits, but the last two (2) options may not, and depending on your life's goals that may be better for you, if you want more control over your work time.

The P.R.N. means, as necessary, where you arrange with your employer the times you are available to come to work. For example, if you would like to work for twenty-four (24) hours per week or month, then you divide that time into their shifts-schedule: eight (8) or twelve (12) hour shifts.

Challenges and Your Future in Nursing

You should be aware that no industry is perfect, and that includes nursing. The challenges in the nursing field include "**nursing shortages**", facing '**burn out**', and new **corporate changes** or mergers that **can affect one's job conditions.**

Where do you see yourself working once you decide to do nursing? Your decisions should be based on your personal strengths and clinical experience. You will need to read up on your state's laws which vary by nursing credentials. **Remember the rule of thumb is to stay within your own nursing lane or LVN/LPN scope of practice, and do not veer off track.**

The nursing field offers many opportunities to use your nursing education, other than being an employee or independent contractor. You may need to start off as an employee to gain experience and build sufficient clinical skills, to generate income to use as capital to invest in a business of your choice. You should have at least two (2) years of clinical, bedside nursing experience before branching out as an Independent Contractor or Travel Nurse. I will discuss this further in my second, upcoming book.

Let us consider why you need to control your work life, especially in any job that is highly stressful, such as caring for sick people. Healthy levels of stress are normal, but if you are a nurse with a stable position and overworked, what benefit is that to you or your family? Do you want to be surrounded by material wealth but be in a constant rush to bathe, eat and sleep?

I hope you see yourself as your Creator designed you to be with a plan to take care of your health and personal needs before you can take care of sick or persons with disabilities. You only have this one life to live, so it is important to create balance in your life.

The above situations are not emphasized in detail by other sources of information in preparation for L.V.N./L.P.N. school. Therefore, this book is different in that it will educate you about the issues that affect the money you are about to spend to attend LVN/LPN

school. I need you to start imagining a vision of how you are going to recoup that money, upon graduation!

Modern day living requires us to have a steady cash flow to pay our bills, sustain our dignity, to avoid begging others for help, and to live a well-balanced life to be mentally sound! Always remember that fact as you plan to spend your hard-earn money on any type of education, including nursing!

Therefore, do not look to employers for your job security as you attempt to get any certification or education. In your spare time, use what you know to build your own job stability, even if you are working a full-time job! Play an active role in planning your own job security, even if it scares you, like it did scare me, girlfriend, but I exchanged fear for faith!

Big Vision for Your Life as God Intended

You are better off having a big picture view as you consider becoming a basic nurse with some wise strategies on how to get into a good school. You need to be wise, technologically savvy, and aware of the job market as you plan this new career move!

Therefore, this brainstorming exercise calls for **being an educated consumer before you invest in nursing school.** I am here to help you put together your own plan before you choose which school is right for you! Think about the short and long term(s): three (3) months to six (6) months and twelve (12) to (24) months from now.

To this end, we need the right knowledge, skills, and attitudes to earn our income in this new, artificial intelligence (AI) era where robots will wipe out some jobs. Do you know there are robots that help lift patients, even hug them, and help surgeons in operating rooms? Are you aware that virtual, online medicine-including virtual, onscreen visits are becoming more acceptable in healthcare?

The good news is any nurse will be in demand, because you have a mind and body that machines cannot replace in delivering certain aspects of care. Your homework is to find out which areas of nursing robots cannot replace humans, including you!

Remember you are your own greatest human asset, not your teacher or your spouse or child, or parent, or your pastor, no one can be of service to you unless you help yourself! Therefore, be wise and see yourself as your Creator sees you, forget the non-believers and stick with like-minded, positive people!

The discerning L.V.N./L.P.N. applicant should be informed of the good and challenging sides of choosing a career in nursing. The choice you make today will ensure our patients get the care they deserve, and you get a great return on your own investment of time and money to become a nurse!

Remember, you are valuable to yourself and the nursing profession. **Concisely, I am reminded of Former, President Barack Obama's words, "Be the change you want to see!"**

Nurses as Change Agents!

You are to think of your whole life, and how to balance your daily activities to be physically fit and mentally alert to be ready for school. You want to be a nursing student who can balance your personal life and nursing school.

Therefore, take care of yourself and take time off to get therapy (if needed) or treatment(s) for any wellness issues, before starting nursing school. You must envision yourself having challenges along the way and still thriving, no matter what! I would like you to have a positive, optimistic approach to nursing school!

This book will help shape your world view, and self-image to become a good nursing school applicant. If your personality type is one of empathy, fun, and shared beliefs in the 'beauty of the human spirit', then you are ready for nursing school and the highs and lows of the profession! The good news is the highs exceed the lows, so go for it, run towards nursing school!

Concisely, my book will help you fit your current skills and behaviors to be accepted as a suitable candidate for school! Embrace your small beginning as you

approach L.V.N./L.P.N. school and do not feel less of a person for starting at a basic, foundational level!

Identify Your Priorities

During this planning stage, I encourage you to consider the possibility of becoming a business owner to create passive income while you sleep. **You need to be business minded about any career choice in these challenging times.**

The pandemic was a bad event, families lost loved ones and costs of living increased: mortgage rates, apartment rentals, gas prices, school fees, cars, and medical costs. Salaries remained the same as we tried to rebuild our lives and make sense of the mental confusion and uncertainties of life!

Also, necessities like food: eggs, fish, chicken wings, and other meats have increased in prices, take a visit to your nearest grocery shop to see what I mean. Thank God, I can still afford my groceries at my favorite places: Trader Joe's, Whole Foods Market, H.E.B., Kroger's Walmart, Fiesta, Costco and Sprouts Farmers Market.

While **I can afford to buy my essential supplies at my favorite stores, inflation may cause our favorite places to raise their prices!** Therefore, that situation should motivate us to improve our work skills to increase our earnings to continue to afford our essential needs! **Nursing school can be your own "come up" or "golden opportunity" to afford the kind of life you want!**

Therefore, as you read my book, think strategically about your next career move. Whatever you do, do not quit your day job yet- unless you can afford to do so, because you will need part of your current job earnings to save for school.

Remember, be nice to those who help you on your path, and do not 'break bread' with those who do not support your plans to improve your life. The latter group will hinder your plans and distract you from your goals! Fortunately, there are many supportive, social media groups you can join with people on your level of thinking! Similarly minded, nursing students in your social groups will help you stay focused and succeed in nursing school. Remember, "...with God all things are possible" Matthew 19:26 KJV!

Appreciate your team.

Also, to become a great nursing student, you will need the support of other helpers to give you good recommendation letters, and wise/RN Mentors to advise you (thank you Howard, Edgar, Rodilyn, and JoAnn).

Remember, you will meet nice people, or angels disguised as organizational support, financial helpers, and motivation along the way! Also, **your prospective classroom teachers and preceptors at clinical sites will be your greatest assets, so treat them with respect.**

Likewise, your personal copy of this book serves as a 'Notebook', so feel free to write your notes in the spaces provided. Yes, this book is part journal and planner too!

Chapter 2
Start where you are.

Be wary of people in the profession who attempt to belittle your efforts, for applying to a lower tier educational program, such as L.V.N/L.P.N. I must warn you, there is a rumor on a reputable website that if you do a State, Approved program, you will not be able to sit the licensure/NCLEX Exam to qualify for your nursing license. Please research nursing school information from reliable resources. I like to research on my State Board of Nursing website, which happens to be Texas State!

Do not listen to rumors, listen to the facts presented on your State's Board of Nursing website to guide your educational choices. I am proof that you can graduate from a State Approved program, with an L.V.N./L.P.N. Diploma and get the PN license to practice at a humble level—and work at facilities, as an employee or Travel Nurse! And, be accepted into schools to do your R.N.!

To this end, you should be grateful for your little beginning because it is your first step, so savor your success, as a stepping-stone to a higher title- if you desire! The nursing field has many older, Licensed Vocational Nurses who are twenty (20) years in and have zero desire to become Registered Nurses, so do what will work for you! I love learning so I will be in school forever!

Where are you in your career and life? Are you a mom, dad, pregnant teen, or high school graduate? Let me tell you a little about how I transferred out of work to go to L.V.N./L.P.N. school. Some years ago, I was juggling a few job titles, living from paycheck-to-paycheck, and felt no passion for my job(s)! I felt I had learned all there was to learn, and I wanted something that made me feel passionate and with a salary to match!

Also, I was working as a Patient Care Technician (P.C.T.), and a Substitute Teacher in Fort Bend County, Texas. While I enjoyed being in the classroom, I felt unfulfilled. I had titles-including that of Licensed Chemical Dependency Counselor-Intern but felt incomplete, I felt a nursing title would be more appropriate! I needed a change to reflect my passion for life, peace of mind and earning power!

Likewise, I felt like life had handed me the bad end of the proverbial stick. Sometime in 2019, I begun a second attempt at an accredited, BSN/RN degree program for students with a Second/non-nursing bachelor's, (my first was Social Science). However, my work and personal life balance was not happening, I needed a manageable school schedule, or I was going to physically pass out!

Although I performed well in school, I was not getting enough sleep and I felt tired all the time! I felt anxious and juggled twelve (12) hour work shifts, three (3) nights per week, from 7 PM to 7AM. Also, I worked another job, two to three (2-3) times a week, as a Sub Teacher from 8AM to 4 PM. Oh Lord, it was like living in a personal, private hell and having only four to five (4-5) hours of sleep a night!

Therefore, after five months (5) in my BSN/RN program, I left my prestigious nursing program, to do a lower tiered, 12-month, L.V.N./L.P.N. program. I then set personal goals to have a more manageable lifestyle, with the geriatric population, and higher pay! Imagine the L.V.N./L.P.N. job pays $10,000 more per year compared to the master's degree (in psychotherapy/addictions)!

Switching nursing programs during Covid 19 was one of the best career decisions I made in my entire life! Today, I am a working nurse and life is as good as I envisioned mine would be- very peaceful, well-paced, with adequate sleep and engaging in other productive activities!

Can you relate to my story? Are you happy being a C.N.A. or working beneath your goals or true potential? Are you willing to let go of any situation that is holding you back from going to nursing school?

Be in Control of Your Life

Human beings were designed to live a creative life- look at all progressive societies or read ancient history books, from the dawn of civilization till it ends. We are powerful creative beings, so powerful that technology is mimicking how we think and function, but they are not us!

You were born to be productive by using your skills to provide a product or service to benefit someone else, in this case your future patients. You should **aim for a work life where you can control your time, to enjoy a more peaceful life doing what you love. Another person's materialistic measure of success does not have to be the only standard of success. You get to choose your own measure of success, and nursing at any level is a worthwhile profession!**

Remember, nursing school requires one to be physically fit: practice eating nutritional foods, and do body massages for your tired aching feet, and back! Also, I would like you to be the star in your own life by taking care of your mental health too!

Another thing, in your big 'Life plan' as you contemplate becoming a nurse, put in the plan a yearly vacation or do biannual retreats with friends, to stay mentally fit. Remember, you will earn that trip, and if you need to travel alone, do so.

Remember, 'alone' does not mean you are lonely-especially if you are single, did your hair, nails and looking fine-girlfriend, no matter your age, darling! Yes, I said it, "no matter your age, look your best, wrinkles, or no wrinkles, embrace the real you inside your body temple where the spirit of God lives"! Remember, the promise, "You are of God, little children, and greater is He that is in you, than he that is in the world" (1 John 4:4, KJV).

Self-Awareness- Love Yourself!

Self-examination is the key to unlocking the reason you would like to participate in one of the most demanding yet fulfilling career choices in the healthcare field: Nursing! I have important questions to ask you as you continue reading.

This book is about the relationship between your heart and mind, as well as the relationship of like-minded individuals or nursing students. You can be honest in your mind, no one will know your answers, except you!

What is your name? Where are you from and why are you here? Do you have a healthy sense of who you are? Where do you see yourself one year from now? What skills do you have, and what other than L.V.N./L.P.N. can you do? Who can help you get into nursing school?

Have you recognized your source of strength? Are you a Kingdom Believer, an agnostic or atheist? I am not judging only enquiring to get you to take a closer look at yourself, which is a task most people are afraid to do. Are you afraid to fail or succeed? I was anxious until I decided, what is the worst thing that can happen to me if something did not work out as planned? Well, I would learn a valuable lesson of what not to do, and what works! Therefore, either way, I win, and you will too!

Whoever you are, love yourself, and know that someone must have loved you, to give you the gift of life! I appreciate you, and I am happy you have eyes to see and intelligence to read my book and I say, "thank God for giving my reader a sound mind to understand this book!"

Why do you want to become a nurse and what is your passion? Thankfully, I chose nursing for two (2) reasons. First, I love caring for geriatric patients -after years of working with Seniors, in America. Also, I wanted to earn a 'living wage' to engage in work that brought me joy and continue to participate in other interests. **List your hobbies and picture how you can use one of them to create a side hustle.**

Let us consider our modern society and its impact on our lifestyle, choices, and work. First, the technological and geo-political speeds are so fast paced, that we need to slow down a bit to be able to enjoy our favorite foods, social events, relationships, and families to create balance.

Second, we need to spend less time on our cell phones, to minimize addiction to social media information or drama. You do not need to know everything that is happening on social media, because most of those people are promoting their business ventures or themselves. You should be looking for information that will help you build your own business too!

Third, another reason a person may choose a career with longevity such as nursing, is to be able to pursue that career well into their older stages of life. Therefore, if you become an L.V.N./L.P.N. or any type of nurse, then your knowledge and skills are never lost-unless you retire, change your field or transition! I pray that God spares my life for several more decades, so I can work this gig, because the knowledge and skills are priceless!

Therefore, being a nurse, at any level, you can only win, because you carry wellness information twenty-four (24) hours/seven (7) days/365 days a year, for yourself and others. **The sky is the limit working as a nurse to improve your patients' lives, job skills, income generation, and lifelong learning!**

Notice I brought money into the equation. Do you have a healthy relationship with money? Since Covid 19 happened, and prices went up, we are wise to think about our financial security. We need stable jobs and businesses, with stable earning power as we engage in the business of caring. Remember there is talk of a cashless society and some jobs are being done in home offices. How do you see your work environment as you plan to become a nurse?

Do you know nursing is a business? Do you know to succeed in Nursing you must have good customer service skills, in addition to the clinical skills you will learn in school?

Money Plays a Role in Life

You will invest money to pay for your nursing education, uniform, books, and license. Likewise, you expect to be compensated for the nursing duties you will perform once you graduate.

Also, you are choosing a career that will pay you back the money you will invest for your nursing education! The future will pay you back with regular paychecks to pay off the credit cards, Federal or private loans you plan to use for school fees!

Therefore, **when you write your Admissions essay for your school Application, focus on the humanitarian reasons why you would like to become a nurse. The paycheck will come later, you will always be paid for any job you do. The advice is to write about "being of service to patients and the community". The opportunity to discuss money is the last question at the job interview, where your rate will be the amount that an inexperience, new nurse gets!**

Also, the screener who will screen your application, his or her focus is not on the hefty sum of money you will spend on your education; they are looking for students

with the best character traits for their programs. Likewise, everyone has a job to do, and yours is to present yourself in the most positive light to get into the program!

To this end, you will have to impress your prospective school by meeting all the requirements stated on the application form. The character traits and academic subjects you bring are your statistics to build your Applicant profile.

Also, applications are screening tools to your "likability factors" or your emotional intelligence or how well you will get along with others. Your accomplishments need to shine and shout, "I am the one, pick me!". The screener's job is to screen the pile of applications on his or her desk to find and pick you based on what you have to offer the school, compared to the other candidates!

Therefore, in your essay, show them the value you will add to the nursing profession. You should look realistically at what it takes for a school to provide resources to train you, pay their monthly bills and have a high NCLEX pass rate (which depends on the quality of nursing students, like yourself!).

Likewise, some people do not feel comfortable talking about salaries or money in general, so understand that. **Life is about having balance, and money plays a role in each transaction, from the day of birth till one dies or transitions. Each human being needs money at some** point in his or her life, for pampers, dental care, vision health, medical insurance, and even for "pull ups" in old age.

Also, on your Vision Board or in your Journal-Planner know the expected dollar amount your state pays an L.V.N./L.P.N., this will guide your (future) budget spending. Visit this website: **https://www.dol.gov**. Compare the salaries of new L.V.N./L.P.N. nurses versus more experienced nurses on the above job website, as well on this popular jobsite: **https://www.indeed.com**

Have a Reasonable Answer

The main reason for entering any profession is because you feel it is your calling or career based on your interests or skills set. **You are entering this field because you enjoy caring for children, your sick grandma, or you are a Home Health Aide, Babysitter, Nurse Aide, and you enjoy serving sick, old, or persons with disabilities.**

You must have a passion for helping sick people because if you do not, patients are going to sense your low energy. Remember, most patients are alert to some of the following: their names, situation/sickness, time, and location/place. Patients can discern your true character, so be a person of integrity and take your time to introduce yourself and talk to them like they matter to you.

Nursing follows a Business Model

Long ago, America followed a religious model of care, with free or low-cost services based on Godly compassion. **Today, the American healthcare industry follows a business model, and new nurses coming into the field need to be aware of this business framework.**

The healthcare field is a mixed group of professionals, with their own goals. The group includes nonprofits, powerful lobbyists who lobby Washington/The Capital, pharmaceutical companies, insurance companies, private entrepreneurs and politicians attempting to enable more access to healthcare services for their voters.

Hope you are beginning to see the frame around this big picture of your life as a nursing applicant, student and finally a working nurse! The knowledge you glean from this book will enable you to offer your clinical services, with empathy, following state laws and be fully aware – business minded--that you are participating in a business model! **Remember nursing is a service industry.**

Upon graduation, you will be required to follow your State's Board of Nursing guidance in your interactions with the public. I will keep repeating this point like a stuck audio, because keeping your work activities within your "scope of practice" is to honor your State's Board of Nursing (SBON) ethical rules and other relevant guidelines.

Why do You Want to Become an LVN/LPN?

I am progressing deeper into the reason you would like to become an L.V.N./L.P.N., because school will be challenging, and I need you to be convinced in your soul as to why you want to become a nurse!

Examine your personal reasons for choosing an L.V.N./L.P.N. program over an R.N. program; both positions are Licensed professions and pay very well. I am older and knowing myself is key to being brave to become a basic nurse, with the knowledge that this is not the end goal for me.

You should think along this line, and ask yourself, "what is my end goal in this life and how does nursing fit into my larger, Life's Plan?"

You may be in the same situation I was in a while back, or you are a newly arrived immigrant, or you just got laid off and are contemplating a stable career, and you need information to make up your mind. I am here for you if you believe an L.V.N./L.P.N. is a good option for a stable career, even if you do not like all aspects of it!

Also, I know you will be able to tolerate most things about being a nurse until you figure out how **to find the right fit** to blend with your favorite tasks. I know you will never go hungry if you choose the nursing pathway, even if you work only three (3) or four (4) days a week and get paid Bimonthly or daily pay!

Let us talk about your current work life or career exploration activities as you consider nursing school. I know what it feels like to go job hunting, not landing a job and having to do more, expensive training or get more education to get a "Living Wage".

Also, I know what it feels like to have a dream, draft it on a 'Vision Board' and plan goals around it and not have enough money to accomplish it for a long time! Yes, you will need to persevere like I did to accomplish your goal of nursing school, sometimes under the scrutiny of naysayers or haters!

Yes, I can relate to your feelings of discouragement especially if you are an immigrant or working a low, menial job, because at one time I was in your exact situation! I remember the time when I was temporarily 'Out of Status' (another survival book for immigrants only) and had to work as an underpaid, Home Health Aide. Therefore, I can relate to the very things that might be tripping some of you up as you are contemplating nursing school. You can overcome!

Let me give some examples, to prove to you I can relate. I was stressing and worrying about how to get out of the rat maze of hard work and little pay! I was mentally figuring out how to pay for the entire school package: admission exams, First Aid CPR Card, books, fees, scrubs, shoes, past exam papers, study guides, NCLEX preparation courses, State Board of Nursing background check fees, medical/physical exam fees, vaccination shots/fees, drug tests/fees, lunch/money, and transportation/gas costs!

Yes, I can relate to your feelings of utter frustration, and if I can do it then honey, so can you! **Life happens, and if you want to go to nursing school bad enough, you are going to find a legal loophole-back door, front door, private school, or public school to do it—choose any opportunity—go to the school or research online!**

You will need a few mental or spiritual exercises to psych you up for nursing school! While I worked, I saved, fasted, and prayed like I was Biblical Daniel in the Lion's Den of underemployment and low pay!

I am a believer in Jesus Christ's teachings, so having faith is part of my process to figuring my way out of any difficulty! I can honestly say, "I could not do nursing school without having faith in God".

Therefore, I spent some time praying and fasting to be able to make it to the winning side! Remember some physical situations are like difficult stains, and you will need prayers like spiritual bleach to fade them out of your life! The prayers were my soul's cries to God to create a way for me to be able to save enough money to go to nursing school! Today, I am living proof, that God sends answers through ideas and inner soul whispers! The entire process took a few years because I had to work out some personal situations for things to flow, but the LORD Almighty did it for me!

Therefore, I am passing on my own individualized version of what I think can help you once you are determined to go to nursing school through any portal of opportunity! The question is are you ready to accept this information, and customize it to suit your needs regardless of the current obstacles you face?

Are you prepared to Act?

If you are reading this page, then you are ready to take serious action to seize an opportunity to enter LVN/LPN school! Somewhere in your state, in a home or office, or job, there are thousands of readers- reading this exact material, exactly where you are, contemplating nursing school, and they may be one of your future classmates!

Likewise, you will need a little bit of "faith like a mustard seed" (read Matthew 17:20 KJV) to activate you to take the bold step to claim your seat as a student in a school! **Remember, you will meet new friends to share the "highs, and lows" of class assignments, studying for tests and to finally get your PN license!**

Chapter 3
You need faith to win!

Yes, dear reader the words written here are my real 'sweat and tears' from my many attempts to go to Nursing school. **Let me add some context to my immigrant story to encourage you if you are an immigrant.** I arrived in this country, for the second time, two (2) decades ago when laptops, cell phones and social media were not as popular as they are today.

To this end, finding career information back then was harder than it is today. Although now research is easier, it is hard to find everything in one (1) place on the internet, so this book helps you with information in one place and my own personal experiences!

What are your current obstacles, especially if you are an immigrant? Today there is more information available about becoming a Registered Nurse as compared to LVNs'/LPNs'. **The myth exists that there is no place for the LVN/LPN. Research any popular job sites on the internet, for example, INDEED.COM, and you will find many job openings for basic nurses or LVNs/LPNs.**

LVNs and LPNs are still in high demand in health and rehab centers (a.k.a. nursing homes), assisted living facilities, hospice care, home health and on nursing

apps (example, Kare Heroes LLC, and Clip Board to name a few). Hopefully, this book inspires more LVNs/LPNs to get trained to work in this rewarding career!

Make Maximum Use of Your Life

You and I have an expiry date on our beautiful lives, and we must plan our lives with faith and trust in a bigger power, who I know as the Living God who gave us life. We are accountable to ourselves, and our Creator for how we live our lives. No matter how many social fads or norms change, a nurse will always have to conform to what the State Board of Nursing sets out as the guidelines to follow.

Do you know of anyone who buys land, puts a house on it, and has children run it without any accountability? No, I do not know of any such person on this earth, and this is the same way our Creator expects accountability from us as His kingdom stewards, students, or nurses!

Therefore, the person who created you inside the womb did not leave you out in the world without a thought of how you would spend your time. Our job is to figure out why we are here. Did your parents ever ask you to account for the time or money they provided for you to go to elementary school? Yes, with a report card and occasional parent-teachers' meetings.

Also, if you did well, you received rewards- compliments and a gift. If you did not do well maybe you received additional tutoring, or punishment in the form of a spanking or a 'Time Out' in a corner!

Therefore, being held accountable will always be expected of you, wherever you go in life- until the day of death- and you do know that one's death records will be recorded in some databases on earth and within your Creator's databases at some location- believer or non-believer! If you can believe cell phones can communicate for great distances, without knowing how they do so, then it is not a big stretch to imagine how God can communicate with you through your thoughts right now!

Seeing With Immigrant Eyes

Also, immigrants can relate to the many challenges we face on arrival to our new homeland in this case America, where we experience many cultural shocks. For instance, we experience new ways of being or doing such as: exposure to new foods, religions, social expectations and different races/languages/accents-all good, but still a lot to 'take in', all at once!

Therefore, I can readily identify with those who felt shaken to their innermost cores to assimilate and melt in this new society's "melting pot" of diverse cultures, where Black people are called "a minority" as opposed to "the majority". **Nonetheless, being called "a minority, with an accent" because of my skin color or island background, has not diminished God's breath of** life or God's spirit within me! I would feel lost without my Caribbean ways (example: foods, love of cod fish and green bananas, and British, speech patterns), so I make a mental note to hold onto that part of my authentic self! How about you?

To this end, if you were born in this beautiful, American country-whatever your race, and seeking to improve your life, I can relate to your job concerns. Let us as a society, encourage each other, as go about becoming nurses, **because sickness does not come color coded, or gender based or by religious beliefs- we need each other!**

According to the Bible, in 2 Timothy 1:7 (KJV), "You were not given the spirit of fear, but one of faith, love, and a sound mind!" Therefore, encourage yourself and start moving with one hundred percent (100%), resolute confidence in God's ability to guide you to the nursing school of your dreams! I did so and look where it got me!

Stay Positive-Take baby steps.

Therefore, I am encouraging you to go after your goals, even while other life situations are pressing you down. Remember life is difficult no matter where you are on the face of the globe, so be positive, **because every problem has an unseen benefit.**

The solution to our problems may not be what we expect, but there is a right solution to each person's problem! You have decided to research nursing schools and that is a good start. I know the finance to pay for school may be the hardest part to get, so take your time, work, look for free grants, take a low interest loan, or max out your credit cards—it is worth the investment!

You need to have some faith in yourself, do not base your decisions only on what Covid 19 did to the economy, or what the news media is saying. **Make your decision to go to nursing school based on the big vision that God has shown you in your mind or secret place about your life!**

To this end, since God created you, and He has a plan for you to get the money to go to school. You must figure out if this is the right time to go to school based on the available money you have, and how to save more.

Be brave, take notes from my book, and devise a plan to go to school, even if it scares you! I was scared too, yes, I was terrified after many unsuccessful attempts to finish what I had started around 2015.

Also, in 2019 when I decided to step down from my BSN/RN program to go to an L.V.N. school, some sceptics asked me, "Rose, why are you trusting that cultural group for your nursing education?"

I answered, "Thankfully, my school is on the State Board of Nursing website, so I am going to apply!". The most important factor is not look at the faces or culture of the school family, **pay attention to whether your school meets the State Board of Nursing's 'Approval List' to educate you! Remember diversity is beautiful.**

Therefore, it pays to do your due diligence and go online to view your State Board of Nursing website and see which L.V.N./L.P.N. programs are legit. I am a nurse today because I researched schools and chose based upon the guidance of my State Board of Nursing before I wasted hard earned money and time on the wrong school!

I hope my book helps you to pick what makes sense for your situation, to make a wise decision. If you are afraid of failing, do not let fear stop you; the schools usually recommend resources to help you do better. You have nothing to lose except your fears, which you can substitute with faith and move in the right direction! I did it and so can you!

Where do LVNs/LPNs Work?

Also, in my humble opinion and experience, there will always be a place for a basic nurse or LVN/LPN. The work environments in which you will find LVNs/LPNs are numerous including Skilled/Rehabilitation Care Centers, Assisted Living Home Communities, Corrections, Home

Health, Hospice, Substance Abuse Centers, Insurance Companies, a few hospitals, and Outpatient clinics.

LVN/LPN Duties

This knowledge is "the big scoop" for a prospective nursing student: **your clinical duties as an LVN/LPN will depend upon your scope of practice or State's Board of Nursing rules**. For example, some of your basic tasks will include administering injections, breathing treatments, changing colostomy bags, Bolus/G-Tube feedings/dressings, wound dressings, taking and fulfilling doctor's orders, hanging an IV treatment, measuring urine from a foley/supra pubic catheter, Glucose monitoring/giving insulin injections, and many other duties within your scope of practice.

Remember if you work as an LVN/LPN **your work environment determines who will supervise you**. For example, if you work in a clinic your supervisor may be a Nurse Practitioner or Medical Doctor or Dentist. If you work in a nursing home your supervision would be by a Registered Nurse, such as your Director of Nursing, but you will take doctors' orders from the Primary Care Physician.

Chapter 4
How do you get ready?

You may have questions as you contemplate going to nursing school. You should separate fact from fiction and know the difference between the duties of your current job, especially if you work as a Certified Nurse Aide (C.N.A.) versus that of an LVN/LPN.

Sure, if you are a Nurse Aide, Medication Aide/Tech, or an office Medical Assistant you have collaborated with nurses, you see what they do, you even feel you can do their work with your eyes closed! **But are you licensed to do it? Nursing is a licensed profession in any of the fifty (50) states in America, and beyond its' shores. Therefore, stop wishing and get ready for school!**

Should You Work While in School

Preferably, if you can afford to, you are better off not working, because your time will be fully focused on school. Likewise, if you are married or live with other family members, where who pays the bills is an option, you all can agree who works while one of you attends school. Marriage is a team effort, especially if one must undertake nursing school, with children, a spouse, church life, school life and work life. Planning is essential, discussions as to who does what, when, and how, need to be addressed before school. Remember this is a commitment of nine (9) to twelve (12) months, depending on the length of the program.

Sometimes you may make a wrong move in choosing a nursing school, but do not give up, learn from a false start, and keep trying. Let me give you a personal story, in early 2015, I was accepted in an LPN program, in Long Island, New York. The school offered me a loan package of $11, 000, alongside my personal deposit of $4,000.00 to start school on September 4th, 2015. Unfortunately, I had a sick family member, so I made the dreaded decision of overstaying my August 2015 visit, to care for my dad overseas. Although the decision caused me financial, relational, and emotional losses, I have never regretted spending more time with my ailing father then!

Meanwhile, the nursing school was not empathetic of my predicament, not at all, it was all business! I lost $700.00 of my $4,000 deposit, because of 'administrative, processing fees to hold the seat'. Can you believe I was refunded only $3,300.00 of that $4,000 deposit?

Although I provided a letter from one of the doctors who cared for my dad to prove I was a caregiver for my sick father, that nursing school had no heart to give me a break! **Remember, I told you the U.S. healthcare** system follows a business model, so take your feelings or emotions out of the equation, factor in the money you will spend on your education and take well calculated risks to get into school, work hard and recoup your investment! Remember, what this older woman is saying to you younger folks out there-life is tough for everyone, so do not leave yourself out of the overall picture.

Fortunately, God in His divine providence led me to another opportunity several years later! Therefore, let my experiences inspire you to not give up, even if an opportunity seemed missed, there is a plan for your nursing life! Also, nothing on planet earth can stop God's plan for your life because it is His desire to give you the desires of your heart as one who has a relationship with him (Psalm 37:4).

You should carefully observe what worked for me, and what did not, and use only the things in this book that can help you create a great plan for yourself. The choices you have right now may seem limited, but you should act on the things that are within your control. For example, if all you can do now is get information, then collect information, then take a drive or walk or a train ride to visit schools. If you take one step closer to your goal, one day you will cover all the steps or actions to become a nurse!

Also, I am aware students in some schools did not work while they attended nursing school. Fortunately, they had saved some money before, while others got help along the way, as their programs progressed. Personally, I worked for a while when I started LVN/LPN nursing school, but several months later, I had enough funds to stop working to focus on school.

I think if you work during school, you should consider the type of job tasks, versus the amount of time you will need to allocate to study, to do class assignments and sleep! For example, if you work as a Home Health Aide, you can attend school in the day and work some nights per week. Home Health Aide, CNAs, Hospital Transporter, Uber Driver, stocking shelves, Pharmacy delivery, Night Lab Techs or food delivery are some examples of jobs you can do while you attend nursing school.

Also, if you decide to work, check out your class hours, is your program a hybrid program of onsite classroom visits, and online sessions? Is it morning sessions or afternoon sessions or both, and how many days? Whatever it is, arrange your work time, in blocks of days or nights, three (3) times maximum per week, based on your class schedule. You are better off not working, but in the real world you may have to work to pay your school fees!

What Kind of School Hours Do You Want?

Some community/state schools have hybrid programs where you can go some days, and on other days stay home to do online assignments. For instance, I know of a student who attended her LVN/LPN program at a Community College in Houston, Texas, twice per week, and found time to work two (2) nights per week. Luckily, she had family members to help her with some money to pay for LVN/LPN school!

You will figure out what to do, based on your situation, I am only offering suggestions on how to find ways to go to school. You should **set aside a minimum of (3) hours daily to study and do assignments for you to be successful in class work, homework, and weekly tests. Therefore, you will need a total of fifteen (15) hours of Study Time per week to commit to all your subjects, usually an average of four (4) subjects per quarter or every three (3) months).**

Whatever you decide, **do what is right for your situation, do not listen to the doubters who say, "do not work". I know some younger immigrants (between ages 21 to 40 years old) who worked and faced a harder set of circumstances as they successfully completed nursing school!**

Some of us must work; it can be the best and worst of times, if you are single, with no one to help you. The advantage of being single is you have no one to distract your focus, so that allows time for peace, sleep schedule, work times, study times and school hours. The disadvantage of being single is you are on your own providing for yourself!

Also, another reason some people must work while they attend school is they do not meet eligibility requirements to get certain types of state assistance: food stamps (for basic groceries), help with housing, or free health insurance (e.g., Medicaid for the indigent poor). Fortunately, there are state scholarship programs that you qualify for (last chapter), so plan, save your money, set your alarm clock, and achieve your goal!

Therefore, do what is right for your situation! I managed to start and finish nursing school, as a single woman, and look where hard work got me today! I survived the alone times and overcame the temptations to procrastinate on assignments. **You will win in the end. The right mental attitude, financial preparation and readiness are your secret strategies to completing nursing school!**

You Need to Prepare Months Ahead

If you have begun your preparation to enter a private, LVN/LPN Career school, and you have your school fees, you will need a minimum of sixty (60) to ninety (90) days to fulfill the obligations of your Application Packet. **Create a list of your potential schools and visit them to have a mental imprint of your intention on each school.**

For example, I visited a popular, private school in Katy, Texas, with a Financial Aid program, and another private school (without the FAFSA), but I chose the latter school in Richmond, Texas because it appealed more to my situation: it costs less gas to fill my car, cheaper tuition costs -at the time, and met other requirements for my life!

Therefore, an initial visit to the school you plan to attend is especially important, for **by visiting the place you will get a feel for the place, where God will allow good people to help you gain entry**. I visited my school three (3) times before I made up my mind to attend! **The third time I visited, I met a welcoming staff member, who turned out to be one of the owners, and she ensured the Administrative Assistant gave me a tour of the entire school to see if I liked the vibes.**

Fortunately, I was happy with the visit. I was provided with the school's Admissions' Requirements: application package, name of the HESI textbook, and how to practice for the test. I felt empowered by the school, so thirty days later I had studied the test material and was ready to do my Admissions Test!

Therefore, I hope you feel encouraged by my tidbits of information and do not give up, no matter your obstacles! Let me share another example of perseverance, one time, I had applied to an RN program at a Community College in Texas, before attending my BSN program and later the LVN school.

Although I had met all scholastic requirements, I received an email which stated "...you met all requirements, but we only had 30 seats with 124 applicants, you will be placed on a Wait List, but you will have to redo HESI after 12 months". Can you believe that school? I think they should have stopped collecting applications and fees after sixty (60) applicants to prevent others from wasting time and money!

I took that experience as a test of wits, and did not give up, and God in His wisdom, worked behind the scenes to have me visit another school, at the right time! **You must keep your intentions and goals clear in your mind as you 'battle' unexpected situations and claim the promises of God to get admitted, it is His 'Battle!' (2 Chronicles 20:15). Therefore, your only job is to believe, pray, and take the right thoughts that come into your mind to take decisive actions-because nothing happens without taking physical actions in the natural world!**

You Will Win

Your decision to go to nursing school is an announcement to God Almighty, that you want this nursing education, and you have taken a step in the right direction. The Lord, **Jesus Christ says, "...knock and the** door will be opened, seek and you will find, ask and you will receive" (Matthew 7:8 KJV). I believed those words, and you must believe in your Creator's power, if you are seeking to attend a legitimate LVN/LPN school!

Therefore, I have a few more questions for you as I write, and the first is: **what does your school need to fulfill entry requirements?**

What are your school's Entrance Requirements?

The school I attended wanted passing scores in some subjects on the **HESI Admission Assessment Exam Review Test.** This was my initial, Admissions or **placement** test.

Some schools may ask for prerequisites in science subjects like Anatomy and Physiology or they may offer it as part of your nursing curriculum. **Find out everything your school needs before you sign off on the dotted line or commitment letter.**

Most schools require you to have these basics: money for school fees, high school diploma, entry exam pass, prerequisites, a five (5) or ten (10) panel drug screen (urine or blood test), some vaccines, American Heart Association CPR card/renewable every 2 years, and a yearly, Physical/health report. **Congratulations on starting the application process! Remember to finish what you started!**

Nursing will improve your life!

You can do it, just like I did! **You have something extra to guide you which I did not have, this book with my own hardships and success! I wish someone had authored this book to tell me what to expect and how to deal with specific situations, people, and rules of life before I went to nursing school!**

In retrospect, I did many certifications (including nursing prerequisites, immigration paralegal) and had a master's degree **before I made up my mind to become an LVN/LPN. Later, upon LVN/LPN licensure, I had more job fulfillment and made more fast money than with any other positions held in the United States of America!**

Sometimes, you are juggling a lower paying job as you are considering improving your job skills. For instance, when I was a Substitute Teacher in 2016, with a college degree, I made about **$125.00 USD for eight (8) hours per day, compared to an LVN/LPN who spends less time in school and makes a minimum of two hundred dollars ($214.00 USD) per shift, for the same eight (8) hours.**

The basic nurse who works a twelve (12) hours shift, can make between $330.00 (employee rate) to $545.00/Premium rate (with Agencies as Independent Contractors or Travel Nurses)! Hope you are paying attention to your potential earnings as a wise, career-oriented nurse!

How The Pandemic Affected Us

The Covid 19 pandemic changed my entire outlook on the job market and life in general. Research shows that artificial intelligence (AI) is a new technology that will positively impact a lot of new jobs. You can be part of this exciting new frontier-where new technologies will mimic every action or activity imaginable, with innovative platforms, to share what you know, with the people who need the exact information, product, or service you offer. Let us harness the benefits of this new technology with responsible right actions to heal and not hurt!

Think a year or two ahead, tell yourself that upon graduation, you will have a normal life, and daily rest. **Also, make and keep some promises to yourself. First promise, you will create a simple business plan, as a backup plan should another pandemic affect your normal job routine. Second, promise yourself that you will get in the habit of learning to sit still, quiet your mind from the day's events, rest, and focus on the actions necessary to start your side hustle to build passive income, while you sleep!**

I became an LVN/LPN beyond my 50th birthday. You may be younger than that or older, and whatever your age, you must take a chance on you! I know you can do

it if you start one action, it will lead to another step, until you take all the necessary steps to get there! Count your blessings of sight, smell, touch, sense, hearing, taste, and discernment among other qualities to help you move towards nursing school.

You are reading the book of someone who overcame all kinds of challenges to remain authentically herself/by choice, with behaviors and thinking customized to "blend in" with American culture! To this end, I experienced a lot of the same challenges or pressures that some of you are going through right now; **I did my best with the little I had and left the rest alone. I focused on the things I could control and ignored the rest!**

Let us examine typical scenarios faced by immigrants. You are trying to make the six (6) points to get your Driver's license, but you are missing one (1) point, or you are working a menial job below your education and skills and must settle for whatever is available, to survive.

You may be facing ridicule from a few folks as you work a menial job to save for school. Permit me to quote from a wise woman, **Accomplished Concert Artist, Fashion Icon, First Black Miss America, and Actress, Vanessa Williams who once said, "Success is the sweetest revenge!"** Vanessa was stripped of her crown but lived to get an apology 30 years later, from the same organization that stripped her of that crown!

You need to have a plan to avoid negative people at all costs, because they will drain your energy and peace of mind! You need to choose to become your best self and be your own best friend-like I did, no matter what!

Let me tell you how I built strength and tenacity over the years to be my own best friend. **I make it a practice to hide and dodge negative vibes, including negative people at work, church or anywhere- I run away from them like bees are chasing me!**

Life has challenges. The Good Lord knows that life is about focus and takes mental energy to be consistently positive and optimistic! **Therefore, for your own peace of mind, avoid any person, situation, or place that will distract you or make you lose focus on your goals- and feel free to block them on your social media accounts!**

Also, I stayed resolutely focused and positive! **The only difference between where I am and where you are is what you do with the time you have left-after you read this book!** You and I have exactly twenty (24) hours in a day, multiply 24 hours by three hundred and sixty-five (365) days, to calculate the number of hours you have per year to get into nursing school or to start a business!

Fortunately, my LVN/LPN journey has a successful conclusion, and I would like the same for you! Therefore, I would like you to be resilient, focused, and tenacious like a Biblical, warm blooded, harmless dove and as wise, as a cold blooded, reptilian serpent

(Matthew 10: 16, KJV). **Also, I would like you to get inspired by reading my self-help book, "Becoming Bright: You are the Three Billion Genetic Blueprint!" (Https://www.Amazon.com).**

Notes

Write three (3) character traits that you possess that will enable you to become a great nurse?

Chapter 5
You are not alone.

Y ou are not alone in life. The road of life is full of fellow travelers, same as students in nursing schools in the United States of America. You will meet new people, some will be your friends, and others will decide to constantly compete with you, for no reason at all! Whatever the situation, stay focused on your goal, especially if you belong to Almighty God, and you will surely overcome and succeed in nursing school!

This book is valuable to you as you move from where you are in life towards taking specific steps to enter nursing school. If you have a prayer life with God above, then I know you have a beautiful mind, with passion and tenacity to achieve your nursing diploma and license!

It is okay to be nervous.

I know how nerve racking you may be feeling to take that giant leap of faith especially if you are short on time, money, and energy. Let me give you a big, comforting, air hug to build your inner strength and for courageously going after your dream! **I am proud of you**

for making the decision to upgrade your skills to improve the lives of patients and your own!

Permit me to share a few of my deepest, intimate feelings before I became an LVN/LPN student. I experienced some anxiety and kept changing my mind several times each time I applied to an LVN/LPN school. I had fears about the risks involved in choosing a lower tiered program, compared to the gold standard of a BSN/RN for a Second-degree holder (who I am), but I wanted to be less burdened with both school and work.

Likewise, I was older, compared to younger students, and I was thinking about long range plans for retirement. I was considered a non-traditional student – but luckily, I did not feel out of touch, nor did I allow any negativity to discourage me! **Can you imagine where I would be, had I allowed my anxious feelings or negative opinions of others to stop me from accomplishing my dream? If that had happened, I would not be here writing this book to teach you how to accomplish what I did!**

Consequently, I know fear was my biggest obstacle before I grew in faith. Sometimes you must be afraid and take positive actions! **I acted brave until I felt brave! I wrote a list of things I needed to do, I worked so hard until I sprained my right wrist! I told myself, "It is do, or die", as I completed each task, I checked them off, and applied! I must confess, it was mentally draining at times, but getting into school was worth all the** anxieties, because it meant I stood a chance of finishing what I started- and I did finish, and you can too!

The Living God worked out every challenge- **the biggest challenges were getting the money to fund my education, buying gas, food, and paying my monthly bills-while in school!** I grew bold in faith, about what I wanted, and when I did not have all the answers, **I watched YouTube videos of Motivational speakers like Les Brown, who said "You got to be hungry, for what you want in life!"** Hilarious to hear him say it, and so true!

Likewise, I read great books, including the Bible- **I took whatever good advice that was helpful and ignored the tips that did not apply to my situation.** I know you may feel a little anxious like I did, so you are a normal person, we are all scared when faced with new or intimidating situations. **The thing to do is initially get quiet about your plans, and only share with one (1) or two (2) people you trust or go it alone, optimism helps one get far in life.**

Additionally, I exchanged FAITH for FEAR, and fear is "Forget Everything and Run or Face Everything and Rise, the choice is yours" (credited to Zig Ziglar, 2017). **I simply believed in myself as a Child of God, and I moved in the direction of my unshakable belief in God's ability to assist me, and He did!**

Take a Chance on You

Be scared, but act, take one step at a time, until you complete all the necessary steps to become a Licensed Professional Nurse (LPN or LVN)! I did it, and you can too!

Some days, prayers and the action of fasting were my only strategies! There were times I felt overwhelmed by the many assignments! I found comfort playing spiritual songs by Gospel Artists: Tasha Cobbs (Break every Chain), Yolanda Adams (The Battle is the Lord's) and Jekalyn (Bigger) to ease my troubled mind. **I felt frustrated, but I stuck to the dream! I never gave up, and you should stick to the dream and not give up too!**

Truth be told, one day, I felt so overwhelmed with paralyzing mental fear because of a messenger of doom, that I sat on my sofa and bawled like a baby. I had a good therapeutic cry, which was good for my soul, and continued my schooling like nothing happened. Later, I was able to afford the luxury of not being in the same social setting with that negative person, and poof I was gone! Remember your peace of mind comes first.

Therefore, remember my stories when you face your Goliath moments, as a person or situation, which may threaten to stop you from completing nursing school. Now, listen to me, "Cry, crawl, pray, believe you can, remind yourself even if you feel like dying, you won't die, and you are not giving up on your goal!"

Trust me, when a woman like me acts "good crazy" as if I have nothing to lose, as I shower my atmosphere with God's words to shield me, even the negative cloud of frustration or depression must lift and drift away! Hope you get an idea on how to push through, even when you feel isolated, remember a 'Child of God' is never outnumbered. The prophet Isaiah reminds us, "There are more with us than they that be with them"2 Kings 6: 16-18).

Some days you will feel helpless, like you do not know what you are doing, because some courses are challenging. Luckily for you, my next book will give you all the tips, tricks, and strategies you will ever need!

Do you get the mental image of how committed I was to finishing nursing school? I was 'all in, locked in", like I was on fire, I was passionate about what I wanted, and I did not care who thought I was weird for believing in myself at my stage and age in life! I am a living testament that "good crazy always gets good results". Yes girlfriend, this is my own made-up, personal quote in the heat of personal battles. Good results await you!

How far have you traveled to get to your decision to go to nursing school? I am guessing it was not easy. Also, if you are fresh out of high school it may feel normal or different, but you too can make it! **I traveled a long way**

mentally in my heart and mind to arrive at nursing, and I have no regrets, so take courage!

Also, I know many other students who were in other fields such as: teaching, banking, computers, construction, emergency services and accounting before they chose nursing. **We all need to start somewhere to get into nursing!**

Nursing school attendance is about good habits, discipline, and focus. Make an inventory of your current likes and dislikes about yourself, your friends, and places where you spend your time. For instance, I started out as a college educated Teacher in my first career, in my twenties (20's), on a Caribbean Island.

Consequently, I had soft skills or emotional intelligence, and discipline that transferred well into the nursing field. Moreso, I loved old people, and working with geriatric patients is like a dream come true! I love meeting Seniors in their eighties (80s) who talk about how they lived their lives, and the nuggets of wisdom they learned along the way! The information I gain from those who are alert and oriented, is priceless for my own personal growth! Life is a cycle of interactions we can learn from.

Therefore, use my stories as your own templates to weave your path or lane to take the necessary steps to enter nursing school! Also, assess your current, transferable job skills that you can use in nursing school.

The short end of the above story after teaching in my homeland, I was upgraded to a few public service positions and was able to gather a lot of information about what kind of jobs I enjoyed. I had a list of things I was good at, for example: writing and computing skills to do work assignments, and right now I am using those skills. Also, I knew I needed a change of environment to celebrate living life on my own terms, thank God for giving me the courage to make that happen!

You need to do the same inner exercises above, reach into your memories and make notes of your positive behaviors, skills, experiences, and wisdom to apply them to new opportunities that come your way! **What looks impossible, is possible with God, (Matthew 19:26).**

Chapter 6
Think like a businessperson.

This book is written at a basic level for High schoolers and career-changers who would like to get into nursing for love of people and stable earnings. Also, for your safety and protection as a nursing student you are required to do annual vaccines: such as Flu and PPD- skin tests or chest X-ray plus frequent Covid testing to remain employable. Also, upon licensure, periodically (every 24 months or so) you will need to keep your license up to date, by doing some Continuing Education Units (CEUS).

I think this chapter will save you a lot of frustration later in your career if early on you realize nursing is a service-oriented and hospitality-type business! The work environment, like nursing school, is a smaller reflection of the wider society, with great team players, and some who are indifferent- stay away from the last group!

In summary, I need you to get a feel for the new activities involved in your decision to become a licensed nurse. Most importantly, what is in it for you, your school, your patients, or clients? What is in it for the corporate investors or your employers who own the facilities or nursing homes, or health insurance companies, or agency who will put you on the job? Think of your responsibilities and rights as you plan for this important career as an **'at will' employee, a unionized one or an Independent Contractor with personal liability insurance.**

What kind of nurse will you be?

You have some critical questions to answer for yourself in this chapter. Let us expand on the above question. Do you want to own a school that trains Certified Nurse Aides or LVNs/LPNS? Do you want to own a business that helps tutor LVN/LPN graduates for NCLEX PN Review and exams?

Do you want to be a test writer at one of the reputable test writing companies to prepare nursing students for exams? You may want to own a Personal care Service to house veterans or a Home Health Agency to service clients in their homes. Do you want to work in Dermatology, alongside a doctor**? Where do you see yourself after you get your license?**

Most importantly, **I need you to understand, while you are contemplating nursing school based on your compassion for others, it will always be a business in America! Therefore, think and plan strategically, like a businessperson.**

Also, the life experiences of an older woman or one's life expectancy rate may inspire a separate set of choices as compared to a younger highschooler or career changer, age 18 to 45 years old. Therefore, if you are in my age group you must take into consideration some basic questions:

"Do you have the stamina, mental tenacity, patience, perseverance, and physical well-being to work with sick, mentally impaired, or aged persons for two to five (2-5) days a week? Can you lift, shift, or reposition at least fifty (50) pounds-whether it is a person or medical equipment?" How would you react to negative people in the workplace?

The answer to the last question is important: by upgrading your education, skills, and marketability in the field to be among high level critical thinkers! The last option is a good reason for you to consider becoming a BSN RN level nurse, if you have a choice and the money to pay for that option!

Therefore, you must plan your career based on your age, health, mental stamina, Life Plan or mission, and stage in life. Your needs may be different from mine in this phase of your life, so do what is right for you, and you will win- because destiny has willed our lives in seasons or timing that is right for each one of us!

Notes

Write a list of five (5) ways your life would improve if you became a nurse.

Chapter 7
Who makes up your Health Care system?

G et to know your **State Board of Nursing (SBON)**, this board is important to get into nursing school; once you graduate your **SBON** will keep you updated on the rules governing your license, and continuing educational requirements. **The SBON keeps the public safe, informed, and it is vigilant against imposters.**

For instance, **The Texas Board of Nursing publishes a bulletin four times a year: January, April, July, and October to keep nurses informed of the current news, issues, and guidelines in nursing.** Schools, nurses, nursing accreditation bodies, private and public officials all hold their State BONs in high esteem, and you should too!

Nursing is part of the Healthcare Industry

According to healthcare analysts, McLaughlin & McLaughlin (2015), America's healthcare system is comprised of: **for profit big corporate firms, nonprofits, and lobbyists** to affect healthcare policy, services offered, **distribution of specialties, and staffing-for example, in nursing.**

People pay into the system to get what they need, and others are marginalized and unable to gain access, were it not for **federal or state programs, like Medicare** (Parts A and B) and your State's **Medicaid** for the indigent poot or those unable to work. The discussion is outside the scope of this book, but to be a nurse it is helpful to have a little knowledge of who and what makes up the health care system (*Health Care Analysis, pp.154-173*).

.

Employers versus your BON Rules

Also, you will learn the phrase "first do no harm" as a nursing student. **Your State Board of Nursing is a beacon of light to guide your nursing career.** If you are unsure about a potential clinical/job situation, do not hesitate to check out your State BON's website for the rules. **For instance, in Texas, LVNs should read Rule 217.11 Standards of Nursing Practice to know their scope of practice (https://www.bon.texas.gov).**

Upon completion of your school program, before you do your NCLEX PN exam, you will be required to do your State BON Jurisprudence (ethics) exam. Remember, when in doubt your State Board of Nursing rules supersede your workplace operational rules! You can always get another job, but not another license, so use wisdom at your place of employment!

Treat People Well

You will have the title **"clinician" or "provider of service",** depending on your nursing role(s), after you graduate. The following quote **"Knowledge is power" by Sir Francis Beacon, 1597 is true in all aspects of life, including choosing your LVN/LPN profession and having good customer service skills!**

Life is organized by known/visible and unseen karmic rules or spiritual laws. While you did not make the rules, to be able to win at home, school, recreation, or work life, you need to follow rules. **Thankfully in this book you are being introduced to all the participants and activities involved in the nursing field long before you venture into nursing school!**

Have Good Intentions

This section is brief to **give you an idea of how significant a role you will play in healthcare as you plan for nursing school.** Let us take a brief look at the political influences in our healthcare system, which includes the nursing field.

Former US President, Barack Obama, designed Obama Care or the Affordable Care Act (2010) to provide low-cost health services for those who need affordably priced dental, vision, and medical care/insurance.

Likewise, Former **Governor Romney of Massachusetts (2003-2006)** created a state health care exchange to help citizens get cheaper health insurance. The Federal and State health Exchange programs have enabled cheaper and more affordable insurance plans for Americans.

Media Powerhouse, Philanthropist, TV Star, and public figure, **Ms. Oprah Winfrey used her influence to produce a documentary on, "The Color of Care," (Oprah's Harpo Productions and the Smithsonian Channel, 2022).** I would appreciate if you took some time to view this documentary to understand how citizens may get different qualities of care, and who gets the worst!

Concisely, whoever you are, as a future nurse, at some time in life, you will need care, **sickness is not color coded** and each person deserves access to adequate healthcare services. **How do you see your role as a nurse in this big picture view?**

Your Investment of Money

Yes, let me repeat **money is a factor in all relationships** in life, you need money to provide for your basic needs such as: house/mortgage payments or apartment/rent, clothes, food, education, utilities, and transportation costs. **According to Ecclesiastes 10:19, "Money answers all things".**

I appreciate the Nursing Instructors, College professors, and accreditation agencies (e.g., ACEN), who have willing hearts to educate nursing students, and improve the nursing profession. **Are you ready to go to nursing school to answer, "the call"? Yes, you are ready because you are reading this book!**

God will give you the strength, resources, and tenacity to do this good work in America, because it is the right thing to do! **Nursing, as you can see, is not only about you, but also about how you will work with other healthcare workers.**

Therefore, you are getting into nursing because you are passionate about providing care and comfort to sick, persons with disabilities, seniors or young persons. Also, you are planning to become a nurse in the United States of America because it guarantees you a stable, long enduring, career, and income in any of the fifty (50) states!

Also, wherever you go within the fifty (50) states, your license is transferable by endorsement and a small fee. Moreso, if your state is a member of the thirty-eight (38) Compact states, then your multi-State license is easily transferable for you to work in other member states. **Research the list of States with Compact privileges now, to find out if you reside in one of those places and what are the advantages of this arrangement.**

Major Healthcare Challenges

America ranked last among eleven (11) countries in healthcare performance compared to other countries, such as Norway and Australia (*Commonwealth Fund Report, Mirror, Mirror 2021: Reflecting Poorly,* August 4, 2021). Americans spend more on health care compared to the returns on our investments of money and resources. **Additionally, nursing shortages and closure of residential facilities are other challenges we face.**

Hopefully, with that knowledge, prospective nurses like yourself will work in partnership with other healthcare professionals to produce new solutions to our healthcare challenges. Also**, beyond your LVN/LPN license, you will need advanced nursing degrees to tackle bigger challenges in the healthcare industry! Are you ready? I hope you have a better idea about the nursing field, so you can prepare your mind and heart to get into nursing school within a year or two!**

Notes

- You will use this assignment to collect pictures for your **VISION Board. This is a powerful, psychological exercise that I have done for over 30 years of my life, and it works every time!**

- Buy a large white board from the *Dollar Store* or *Walmart or Hobby Lobby or Michael's Crafts Store* to create a visual/Vision Board.

- Place cut outs or pictures of nurses in your favorite color scrubs.

- Place pictures of Actions or activities that will get you into the school of your choice. Start one activity or action, then another, until you complete all the necessary steps to get into nursing school (getting your school fees is part of the exercise).

- Also, put pictures of what kind of tasks and type of population (babies or adults) you would like to work with upon graduation.

The above psychological exercises will bring your dream closer to your present state of mind and will compel you to take steps towards your future, as the saying goes, "mind over matter".

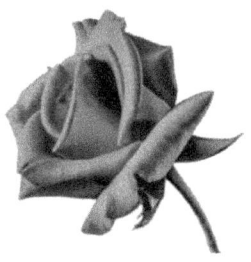

Part Two

Apply to Schools

Chapter 8
Choose a school that fits your lifestyle.

The best L.V.N./L.P.N. school for you is one with a reputation for speedy admissions, and great teachers who train students to successfully pass the NCLEX PN exam to get licensed! Research three (3) schools, assess the things each requires and apply to your top, two (2) schools. Also, **choose the school with the easiest requirements for your situation, like I did!**

Private schools, especially Career or Trade schools, have an advantage of speed of entry into their programs once you meet their entry requirements! Some people find public schools cheaper, but they have limited seats, and are competitive to get in and stay in. I know several people who found success in both types of schools.

Choose the school that works for you. I prefer private schools for the ease, convenience, and speed with how they work. They have no Waitlist! Also, there are many students who graduated from public schools, and are successful LVNs/LPNs too! Therefore, do what works for you, "nursing school is <u>not a one size fits all</u>".

Private Schools or Community Colleges

Some private schools may have weekly schedules of five (5) days, 9 AM to 5Pm, with clinical sessions on a Saturday, each weekend, throughout the school year. Other schools, including state/community colleges may have a hybrid program, where one goes to school a couple of days per week, with in-school classes, and the rest of the week they meet online, then do the clinical portion at a facility, on weekends.

Likewise, some students may choose to remain in their home states or choose to attend a hybrid/online program in another state, for example, Florida. Currently, the Florida BON is reviewing a few schools to see if some programs (with classroom and online attendance) meet Florida's BON educational standards for nursing programs.

Therefore, research your LVN/LPN program before you apply to an out-of-state school online or one that comes to your state and hides behind an LLC entity without getting approval from your State BON. **Remember, many nurses were outed for buying their certificates from fake programs to sit legitimate licensure exams, and now they are out of work, with lower incomes to pay bills and their names are in the news media for all to see.**

Therefore, save yourself from that negative exposure at a fake school because the fake nurse will be demoted, their family will be embarrassed, and the fake nurse will face charges from his or her state of residence.

Fortunately, there are many students who graduated from Approved programs, from Florida and other states. The advice, "Buyer beware" is applicable to any new school you hear about. **Please check your State's Board of Nursing website and if a school is not listed there do not bother to apply, run away, and do not look back!**

Comparatively, **some nursing schools may have you flying or driving out of your city to another city within the same state or out of state, to do clinicals. Please be aware of all the requirements of your education before you put down any deposit**. You may have to add to your school fees: plane tickets, hotel stays, meals, and UBER fares or gas. **Fortunately, there are many students who have successfully graduated from some out-of- state schools and are now working as nurses!**

However, this book is focused on one's home-State, Approved LVN/LPN programs, such as the one I attended in my state of Texas, where one attends a local program, graduates, and passes one's NCLEX PN Licensure Exam.

Also, a note of advice, a state school on '**probation' or conditional status on your State Board of Nursing is still a good school to apply to. To this end, these schools meet certain conditions to be in operation and must follow your state's recommendations for current** student enrollment and improvement during a specific time limit.

Unaccredited Versus Accredited Schools

There are different types of accreditations, for example national, regional, state, employer, and nursing bodies. For this discussion, I need you to research your school and see what type of nursing accreditation and state approval it has. **I need you to choose an LVN/LPN program that is Approved by your State Board Of Nursing.**

If **you choose an Approved nursing program or school that is Not Accredited, you will still sit the same National NCLEX PN exam to get your state's L.V.N./L.P.N. license as those who graduated from Accredited nursing schools!** You need to find out more about the advantages of attending an Accredited school versus one that is State Approved but **not** accredited by a nursing accrediting body. **Remember, the State determines if one is licensed to work as a nurse or not, so if all you expect after school is a license to work, then go where you are able to pay for that education! Research your options and choose what you can afford to pay!**

Accredited schools are all about quality education and meeting certain educational standards set by an accreditation agency (refer to the list in the last

chapter). **Accredited schools have many benefits.** The main benefit of Accredited schools is they prefer accepting Accredited transfer credits from students of similarly Accredited schools.

I attended a school that was Approved by the Texas State Board of Nursing, and since graduating, I was accepted at some Accredited Schools to do my RN program. Also, I am a working nurse, despite online misinformation that you will not get your nursing license to practice if you did not attend an Accredited LPN/LVN school! This is untrue, so be aware of this rumor.

Remember, your State's Nursing Board is the administrative agency that oversees your initial license, renewal, regulates your nursing education (LVNs/LPNs and RNs), visits your places of work, as well as discipline nurses. Therefore, any school that is Approved by your State's Board of Nursing is a great school to go to! Also, employers would like to know if you are licensed by the state board wherever you are applying for your job. Employers can look up your name, find your location and license number in selected databases.

Your life situation may be different from mine, but I have provided you with a lot of information to help you make wise decisions to apply to a good nursing school. **Preferably, if I had FAFSA grants or scholarships and**

was starting fresh out of High school, I would choose any school where my tuition would cost me less without loans. Also, I would choose Accredited schools.

The other reason I would choose an Accredited and Approved school is because nursing accreditation is about the quality and standards set by experienced professionals who know the field. As for being fresh out of high school, I would choose an Accredited program which is also Approved by my State Board of Nursing because new/freshman college students have access to more available free state and federal money, in the forms of grants and scholarships.

Also, grants and scholarships do not have to be paid back, and a fresh man in his or her late teens or early twenties or even thirties would be younger and have more career time to enjoy one's work life over a longer extended period compared to an older worker. Anyway, who is to know how long we have in the field? Therefore, take a chance on you and let God do what only He can do for you, for instance, God can add more years to your life (like he added 15 years to King Hezekiah's life).

Allow Your Immigrant Experiences To fuel you.

Over several years, I spent hundreds of dollars on school application fees, admissions tests, prerequisites/classes, and evaluation reports of my foreign degree to enter various nursing schools in New York, New Jersey, and

Texas. Also, balancing work and school was hard, and I was unaware of an easier way to do so, but recent knowledge about work apps like Kare, Shift Key and Fleet Nurse offer plenty of PRN opportunities for CNAs, CMAs and Nurses!

Also, I went to various school orientation sessions, passed different entry tests, but had some stopgaps to redo prerequisites, after the science ones expired. I was waitlisted several times for several schools for one reason or another. I can laugh at these situations today, but trust and believe they were not funny when I was experiencing the pain of temporary defeat.

Today, I can have a meeting of the minds with you and let you know that if you are an immigrant, then consider yourself lucky with the information in this book. **Prayers, perseverance, patience, and wisdom finally led me to becoming a nurse today. The same can happen for you if you act and move in the direction of your dreams. Some people did not believe in my dreams and discouraged me from pursuing nursing. And where are they now? I can imagine them still talking about a dream and not taking action to get it done! I hope you have the mindset of a champion, and you will go on to achieve your dream of becoming a great nurse!**

Side Conversation with Fellow Immigrants

The immigrant communities in America, have many educated immigrants from all over the globe! I congratulate those of you who have managed to stay employed during and after the unexpected pandemic.

Also, we should all be grateful to God for surviving the pandemic in our right minds! You may fit into one of the following types of workers: Plumbers, Electricians, Construction workers, Babysitters, Housekeepers, Certified Home Health Aides/Personal Care Aides, Computer Technicians, Air Conditioner Technicians, Tutors, Pre School-Administrators, Certified Nurse Aides (C.N.A.), Baby Nurse Aides, Sitters, Data processers, House cleaners and Companions.

Congratulations, if you have managed to take care of your family in the USA, and even managed to spare some barrels of food and clothes to send overseas to your other families back home! Congratulate yourself for having a good heart to help others in times of need!

Also, **I would like to address a peculiar group of immigrants who are working but are not fulfilled, because they have a yearning in their bellies caused by unfulfilled dreams.** I call them 'Unfulfilled Dreamers,' this group may have academic qualifications such as: High school/Caribbean CXC/British "A" or "O" Levels/credits, former Teachers, small business owners, trades men and Crafters. **I am proud of you for having the guts to survive and earn an income after the** pandemic, especially if you are an 'Out of Status' immigrant (many immigrants have overcome that barrier to go on to become nurses!).

I hope you are researching the latest immigration news on how the Federal government is creating legal pathways for **out of status immigrants** in this country. Whatever I know, I plan to share as a Certified Immigration Paralegal. **Disclaimer: I am not a lawyer, and if necessary, I will refer you to a lawyer who is legally trained to answer all your immigration questions. Stay hopeful, continue to stay safe and battle your challenges, until you succeed!**

Side Hustles, other than LVN/LPN

Also, this group has many people with skills to create small businesses related to caring for the aged or something different. Likewise, many have legal status, and are eligible to go to a Trade/Career School to do a Small Business Course. I encourage you to go after your dreams, any dream, such as starting a small, home-based business to sell a product or service, especially during this 'great job resignation'.

Did you know since Covid 19- many workers have reevaluated their lives and how they work, and a huge percentage would like to live their lives differently? Many would like to become entrepreneurs and do home-based businesses- and make money online, away from a boss!

Some people have quit their day jobs and are turning to technology to help them reinvent themselves to use their current skills in new ways to become their own bosses! It is wise not to leave your career planning to chance, and if you have a choice choose to become your own boss.

Be Courageous, Assess Your Options!

Likewise, I am sure there are some of my readers who have skills, for example, in Hair braiding, Nails, Personal Trainers, crocheting for sale or doing Make Up, and can generate their school fees from such activities. Do you know that someone who does hair or makeup makes more money per hour than a new LVN/LPN? For example, I pay my braider $200.00 USD to braid my hair, for three hours (3) worth of work!

Permit me to use the above situation as a teachable moment for you. I worked about six (6) hours as an Independent Contractor Nurse on an App to make that same $200.00 USD to pay her for braiding my hair! I am showing you the 'business-like approach' you need to have if you have similar skills to raise money to pay your school fees! I think raising your own money for school fees beats applying for a loan, with its high interest rates!

Also, I am here to prod you, push you, pull you, carry you, hold your hands, and encourage you to take 'baby steps' toward nursing school or a small business! Whatever you decide, my task in this book is to add

words of wisdom to get you started to do your LVN/LPN program or some economic activity that will yield money. Hopefully, most of you have gotten the message, and the rest of you are contemplating other business ideas- better than nothing, so go to your nearest Career One Stop or Work Force agency and ask for training to start something!

You cannot continue living in a state of uncertainty, without achieving your dream, or else life would seem inadequate and unfulfilled! We survived Covid 19, now we need to re-focus with stronger determination, and with our minds mentally strong, "like flint" (according to Ezekiel 3:9, KJV).

The question is, "Are you willing to put in the time to change the old, negative way your mind works?" I am willing to help you, so keep reading my books and buy my journals/notebooks on Amaon.com for inspiration to start and finish!

Entrance Requirements

Also, if you can answer these questions for yourself, you are ready to get into nursing school! What are the school's entry requirements for the LVN/LPN program you are considering? Which admission tests are you required to sit? For example, is it one of these: ATI/TEAS, HESI, or WONDERLIC? What are the pre-requisites, if any? For example, does your school require: Anatomy 1 and 2, Psychology, Microbiology or College English? Some LVN/LPN programs may have those above subjects built into their program, so take courage and find out.

Also, most **schools do not accept Admission scores that are more than one (1) year old for standardized, admissions tests, like HESI or TEAS/ATI.** Also, some schools do not accept prerequisites that are over 5 or 7 years old. Some private schools do not bother with Prerequisites for their LVN/RN programs, but their price tags are steep, between $30,000 to $65,000.00 USD.

Consequently, my experience in applying to different schools is that some private, nursing schools keep their requirements simple. The schools may ask you for: a high school diploma/GED or foreign school equivalent/transcript, pass a test, ID/Driver's License or Non-Driver's State ID, and Social Security number to prove your identity. And they will ensure you can pay for school and send information to the State BON to give you permission to start school.

The State BON ensures you do not have any Criminal record that stops you from becoming a nurse. **Prior to full acceptance into a nursing program, your school forwards your name to the State Board of Nursing, then they will require you to do a background check. Also, if you pass the IDENTOGO background check, your State Board of Nursing will send you a 'Blue card' in the mail, which is your permission or approval, to begin the nursing program with your school.**

My Preferred Admission/Entry Exams

I prefer HESI to other Admissions Assessment tests, because the practice books were easier for me to understand. There is private, and Community or State Nursing schools that require several subjects on the HESI or ATI/TEAS V, so your assignment is to find out which subjects your school requires you to pass in their test and know the passing score.

Permit me to reference my personal experience with admissions tests. I did all at one time or another in both New York and Texas. However, I am not a fan of some admissions tests. I **prefer HESI Admissions exams and I found the structure of the Admissions HESI easier for my learning style. However, I preferred two (2) other test companies for passing my licensure PN exam or NCLEX PN, which I will tell you more about in my follow-up book!**

Your Learning Style

What is your learning style? Find out how you learn best and use that style to study and pass your entry exams for nursing school. Let me explain what one's learning style may include. I enjoy watching and listening to videos, so I learn better by seeing, listening, and sometimes touching what I see (like in lab classes). **Therefore, watching free videos on You Tube Channels. For example, I enjoyed YouTube videos for students by**

this study resource, 'Simple Nursing,'. I found it a great learning resource for my L.V.N./L.P.N. foundational learning**!**

NOTES

1. Write your State's Board of Nursing information: name, street address, email, contact person, and telephone number. Use information from your State Board of Nursing to find your school or choose two (2) schools to apply to.

2. Write the LVN/LPN pass rates for your prospective school for four (4) years including the current year: 2020, 2021, and 2022.

3. Upon your acceptance, ask your school for the curriculum and each quarter ask for each course or subject outline.

4. Look at the grading system and assignments so you can follow your teacher's work plan to guide your knowledge of the material and to study to be able to pass each course. If there is no course outline, then just follow directions for class assignments.

Chapter 9
Best L.V.N./L.P.N. School in Texas

The best way to check out a school is to read the NCLEX pass rates on your State Board of Nursing website, visit the school campus, talk to past students, read online reviews from former students, and go talk to the staff. Afterall, you will be spending a year or twelve (12) months of your life there, and you want to be fully informed before you go, because life happens!

Also, I chose to attend a Career school, because the program's outline was a perfect fit for me! Likewise, I was impressed with my school's high pass rates for NCLEX-PN, spacious classrooms, and great teachers.

Chose Positive Study Buddies

Nursing school is a microcosm or small part of the larger society in which we live. You will meet good people in life as well as the opposite, and you will attract your kind or type that blends with your personality. I know the person reading this book is a good, decent human being, with ethical, moral, and humane behaviors. We should respect another person's right to be him or herself, whether they follow moral codes that may conflict with ours. Rule of thumb, each person has a right to exist and enjoy his or her life in whatever way he or she decides, and our business is to mind our own personal situations.

Remember, understanding diversity will enable you to have good relationships with new people/lifestyles, genders, new identities/pronouns, cultures, languages, and ways of thinking. I make it a rule to keep my big eyes on my own affairs, to be mentally strong. Therefore, I keep friends closer and a new person at a safe, emotional distance until I know the person better, before I build trust. How about you?

Let us talk about friendships. I believe one should always have four circles of relationships: new people/acquaintances or one's outermost circle in one's life, then teammates- those with whom you work or go to school, then your family and closest friends, who are considered your inner circle. Always use wisdom with each group, especially the outermost circle.

Therefore, choose friends who will support you through good and tough times. Remember to be loyal to those who look out for you. Be a trusted friend, even when you have a difference in opinion because "… faithful are the wounds of a friend" (Proverbs 27:6 KJV).

Remember it is possible to be friendly with some people without being close friends with them. Nursing school can be extremely competitive because human beings have different personalities with different coping styles and behaviors. Also, to be successful in nursing school you will need the help of a few chosen friends. I had three (3) good friends during school, even though we were culturally diverse, different ages, and stages in life. Thankfully, the entire class was a friendly group, and we all did well and are employed!

My LVN/LPN School!

I went to an Approved school in Texas, which is Accredited by business and educational agencies in Texas to train Vocational Nurses. **Also, my school has a strategic advantage over other schools because they work directly with USCIS immigration to help international students who can afford the tuition to come to America to become nurses.**

Likewise, my school is big on welcoming diversity of cultures among students. For example, students were from different countries such as Philippines, Africa, Asia India, China, and me originally from The Caribbean/West Indies. **You would think that with our diverse cultures it was the United Nations in that school!**

If you decide to come on a student visa to the USA for school, do know it is an expensive undertaking to pay for: rent, traveling around, medical/dental/doctor's bills, food, cell phone, utilities, and other expenses. Also, save enough money to take care of your needs because that would be your responsibility if you got approved to travel here for school.

Also, you must follow all the strict school rules that made me who I am as a nurse. The faculty allowed us to participate in prayer for God to guide our success, which is one of the reasons I appreciated my school for its' respect for our different faiths and cultures. **Therefore, I chose my school based on these factors: it accommodated my spiritual beliefs, its' successful L.V.N./L.P.N. pass rates, and the acceptance that I felt from the school family.**

The entry requirements were within my capabilities. The HESI Admissions test was doable, and I passed! The trade school is a HESI testing site, you pay $65.00 USD, to sit the test to qualify for the program- results are same day, so you can have peace of mind!

The school is directed by a formidable team of experts; and owned by two (2) of the best humanitarians I am privileged to know! **The owners were incredibly involved in our nursing preparation; they were at school most days like a real school family. Also, they were "on our case" daily, committed to our education, and there is an "open-door policy" to address student concerns.**

The biggest gesture of 'good will' they did for us during Covid 19 pandemic is that they found clinical sites for us, at a time when it was rare to find places to go to! I appreciated the faculty who thoroughly prepared us for

NCLEX PN licensure exam with almost a 100% passage rate for those who sat the exam and gave us a beautiful graduation ceremony!

My school Accepts Young and Older Students

I wanted to get into a program fast and get out fast, so I went to a simple, LVN/LPN program among students eighteen (18) years to fifty (50) plus! **Therefore, do not allow others to make you feel "less valuable" if you are an older student or an immigrant with an accent, just go with your high self-esteem and 'do you' and mind your own business, like I did mine!**

Likewise, I heard one of my favorite Transformational Coaches, **Lisa Nichols, says, "How someone else feels about you, is none of your business!"** You will need to adopt that thinking each day as you move through life, because you will meet people in life who deliberately attempt to make you feel small- because you are not their version of success. **My school prepared me for success, and I am recommending that you go to my school, if you live in Texas!**

Look up my school's website: **Https://WWW.BellTechCareerInstitute.com.**

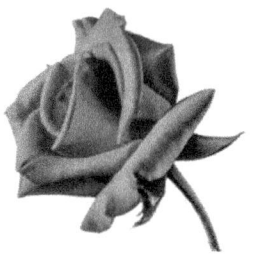

PART THREE
HELPFUL TIPS

Chapter 10
Student Resources

These are my personal ideas on **the ways you can source money to pay for your school** tuition/fees:

- Visit your L.V.N./L.P.N. school, see if there is a Federal Financial Aid program (FAFSA), ask about scholarships, free grants, and your last option is low interest loans.

- I had to use my own private money to pay the $25,000.00 tuition, and I received a $5,500.00 scholarship too, from Workforce Solutions, Texas. The community colleges are half the price of my total tuition, but space may be limited and competitive to get in! The private schools have no waitlist!

- **Visit your State's Workforce Solutions or Career Center in your community to help pay for your LVN/LPN program.** The sum they give is usually based on the annual maximum you can get, for example, $5,500 USD maximum per year. **You must meet eligibility requirements and bring old pay** stubs or bank statements of proof of income for the past three (3) to six (6) months, see if you qualify for childcare payments to help watch your kids while you attend school.

- **Your savings**, from **work (or side hustle)** and family contributions.
- **Grants or Stipends from non-governmental or non-profit organizations.** For example, I knew someone who upon meeting eligibility requirements received a grant to help with nursing school from U.S. Volunteers of America, Texas.
- **Private loans, or credit cards,** for example: Discover Card, Capital One, Bank of America, and Chase. Buyers should beware of high interest rates and do not get cards with an annual fee!
- **Other scholarship help:**
  Careeronestop.org
  Scholarships.com
  Dare-to-Dream Scholarship
  Fastweb.com
  Johnson and Johnson Scholarships

Evaluation of Foreign Transcripts

- Research this website: **Https://www.naces.org** The National Association of Credential Evaluation

Services is an organization of several evaluators, some are more favorable or recognized by your school or employer for job training, school admission or employment. Find out which evaluator your school wants to evaluate your foreign transcripts for their nursing program.

You will need to get a copy of your high school and College transcripts/grades (if you attended college) and their corresponding certificates, to be evaluated by this US based service. Ask your school which evaluator to use, before spending your money on a specific evaluator.

Remember NACES.org is a fee-based service to be paid with a credit card, and call them before you pay online, if you have questions. Personally, **I have used Globe Language Services Inc, based in New York, Educational Perspectives, based in Chicago and Foreign Credential Service of America, Corpus Christi, Texas.**

Schools may ask you to get a Course-by-Course evaluation (costing $150.00 to $200.00 USD) to ensure the foreign education/transcript is comparable to USA credits and a passing Grade Point Average (GPA), between 2.5/C grade and 4.0/A grade. I am happy to report I had over the required 120 equivalent credits to U.S. credits to get accepted into my master's program (I had 135 Credits), so take heart and get your foreign credits evaluated! Also, it is good to know the transferable value.

Additionally, you can evaluate your foreign credits and decide to start over from G.E.D. or High School level, then do so. Also, if you are between 18 to 45 then it is worth it if you qualify for free financial aid/grants, but if you are an older career changer, you will have less time to work with.

Other helpful resources for student preparation:

- **Dress for Success.** This is a national program found in many states, they usually accept you based on a referral from another community or state program, for example, Workforce One Career Center or Workforce Solutions. They help you prepare for job interviews, support your pre-job search, and make you an offer to join the Professional Women's Group, which is an ongoing resource to help you stay skilled!
Veterans and job seekers may benefit from resume preparation, mock interviews, and dressing for the job. **This resource is helpful if you plan to have a job while in school or after you graduate from training or nursing school.**
Personally, I received mock interview preparation from experienced professional women who coached me before my first LVN/LPN job. I am incredibly grateful for this organization and its corporate mentorship of career seekers!

- **Research and know the differences in Scope of Practice for Licensed Vocational Nurses/LPNs and Registered Nurses.** The knowledge will enable you to choose an appropriate program.
- **Know basic Conversion rates** needed to prepare and pass the Math section in your Admissions or Placement Test. (In my follow-up book, I will tell you how I studied for my Math/Pharm class).

- **Know your State Board of Nursing's address and learn its rules governing your nursing program. There are fifty (50) American States Boards of Nursing (SBON);** see if your school is listed on your SBON before you enroll in any school!

- **Know which accreditation agency accredits nursing education programs at different academic levels and see which is relevant to your program. Accreditation bodies:**
    1. The Accreditation Commission for Education in Nursing (**ACEN**), it accredits nursing programs at all levels, starting with practical nursing, diploma, associate, baccalaureate, master's, post-master's certificate, and clinical doctorate.
    2. The Commission on Collegiate Nursing Education (**CCNE**) is the accrediting agency

of the American Association of Colleges of Nursing (AACN); it starts accrediting from the bachelor's level or baccalaureate, then graduate, and residency programs in nursing.

3. The Commission for Nursing Education Accreditation (**CNEA**) was established by the National League for Nursing (**NLN**); it accredits all types and levels of nursing programs: practical, diploma, associate, bachelor's, master's, and Doctor of Nursing practice.

4. The Council on Accreditation of Nurse Anesthesia Educational Programs (**COA**), accredits certificate, master's, and doctoral degree nurse anesthesia educational programs.

5. The American College of Nurse-Midwives Division of Accreditation (**ACNM**) accredits midwifery programs.

Also, when you get into school get your program outline (divided by quarters or semesters) then schedule the program week by week in a planner or calendar. Buy the correct books on your book lists/the most recent editions are best, specific color scrubs, and set your alarm clock!

Remember some LVN/LPN programs are nine (9) to twelve (12) months, so gauge your test taking strategies differently for the types of assignments or tests. You will need to view You tube videos on content, class assignments versus weekly tests versus end of term exams, and lab skills.

Also, I will tell you in my next book how to succeed while in school, and how to pass the NCLEX PN exam, on your first try! I will give you tidbits on how to approach your first job and how to stay focused on learning new skills.

In closing, this is where I end this book and send you a special prayer for God Almighty to give you peace, protection, and safety. **Congratulations to you for choosing a legit nursing school, and hope you find some motivation within these pages to stay focused on becoming a great nurse! And, look out for my follow-up book, "Success Strategies for LVN/LPN school and passing your license exam on the first try".**

Acknowledgements

Accreditation Commission for Education in Nursing (ACEN), Atlanta, Georgia.

U.S. Department of Labor. https://WWW.dol.gov

Former Governor Romney, Massachusetts, USA, _'Health Care Reform_ (2006).

Actor, Media Powerhouse, and Philanthropist, Oprah Winfrey & Smithsonian Channel, _Documentary, 'Color of Care'_ 2022

Former, United States President Barack Obama, _'Obama Care Health Care Reform' (2010)_ and quote, "Be the change you want to see".

Texas, State Board of Nursing. www.bon.texas.gov

Texas Board of Nursing Bulletins, 2022 and April 2023.

King James Bible, Public Domain version.

Mc Laughlin, Craig, and Curtis Mc Laughlin (2015). _Health Care Analysis. An interdisciplinary Approach._ 2nd Edition. Burlington, MA: Jones & Bartlett Learning LLC.

Bell Tech Career Institute, Richmond, TX 77082. WWW.Belltechcareerinstitue.com

Workforce Solutions, Texas. Https://www.WrkSolutions.com

Lisa Nichols, Transformational Coach, quote, _"How anyone feels about me, is none of my business."_

WWW.HESI.com

WWW.ATI.com

2017, Zig Ziglar, quote, "Fear, Face Everything and Rise."

You Tube: Simply Nursing (videos).

https://simplenursing.com

Les Brown, phrase "You Got to be hungry."

Ms. America, Singer, Actress, Fashion Designer, Entrepreneur Vanessa Williams, "Success is the sweetest revenge."

Popular Nursing Apps: Kare Heroes Inc., Clip Board.

Commonwealth Fund Report, Mirror, Mirror 2021: Reflecting Poorly, Aug. 4, 2021

Charles Bon well and Neil Fleming (1987). The VAK/VARK Model: Learning Styles.

United Nations Transforming our world: the 2030 Agenda for Sustainable Development.

https://sdgs.un.org/goals

Https://WWW.bestnursingdegree.com

https://Careeronestop.org

https://fastweb.com

Scholarships.com

Dare-to-Dream Scholarships

Grocery Stores: Walmart, Wholefoods, Trader Joe's, Sprouts, HEB, Kroger, Fiesta and Costco.

Notebooks on Amazon:

<u>For Pet Lovers</u>

Title "Fluffy Stuff, Your Royal Highness Notebook".

<u>For Creatives</u>

"Awesome Light Journal"

"Royal Awesomeness Notebook"

Amazon.Com

<u>For Nurses</u>

"Royal Awesomeness Notebook"

www.ingramcontent.com/pod-product-compliance
Lightning Source LLC
Chambersburg PA
CBHW070650220526
45466CB00001B/377